58 Unique Prostate Cancer Juice Recipes:

All-natural Home Remedy Solutions That Will Get Your Body Stronger and Healthier to Fight Cancer Cells

By

Joe Correa CSN

COPYRIGHT

This publication is designed to provide accurate and authoritative information in regard to the subject matter covered. It is sold with the understanding that neither the author nor the publisher is engaged in rendering medical advice. If medical advice or assistance is needed, consult with a doctor. This book is considered a guide and should not be used in any way detrimental to your health. Consult with a physician before starting this nutritional plan to make sure it's right for you.

ACKNOWLEDGEMENTS

This book is dedicated to my friends and family that have had mild or serious illnesses so that you may find a solution and make the necessary changes in your life.

58 Unique Prostate Cancer Juice Recipes:

All-natural Home Remedy Solutions That Will Get Your Body Stronger and Healthier to Fight Cancer Cells

By

Joe Correa CSN

CONTENTS

ABOUT THE AUTHOR

After years of Research, I honestly believe in the positive effects that proper nutrition can have over the body and mind. My knowledge and experience has helped me live healthier throughout the years and which I have shared with family and friends. The more you know about eating and drinking healthier, the sooner you will want to change your life and eating habits.

Nutrition is a key part in the process of being healthy and living longer so get started today. The first step is the most important and the most significant.

INTRODUCTION

58 Unique Prostate Cancer Juice Recipes: All-natural Home Remedy Solutions That Will Get Your Body Stronger and Healthier to Fight Cancer Cells

By Joe Correa CSN

The prostate is a vital gland in the male reproductive system that wraps around the male urethra. Its main function is to secrete an alkaline fluid that constitutes about 30% of the semen volume. However, prostate problems are one of the most common health problems in men. The fact that one man in seven will be diagnosed with prostate cancer is simply surprising. This extremely serious disease is the third leading cause of cancer death in the US. These statistics suggest that taking care of your reproductive health and recognizing the symptoms of prostate problems is vital for preventing these complications.

The most common symptoms of prostate problems and cancer include urination abnormalities, pain, painful ejaculation, pelvic or abdominal pain, erectile dysfunction, extremity swelling, and blood in urine or semen. Although not all of these symptoms indicate prostate cancer, they might be a sign of some serious medical conditions that require an immediate medical intervention. Prostate cancer can only be diagnosed by tissue biopsy.

The question is what can you do to prevent prostate cancer? The answer lies in a proper diet. Our body is a truly fantastic organism that has the ability to defend and cure itself. This is why it's crucial to help your immune system to get stronger and boost your overall health.

Eating the right amounts of fruits and vegetables will definitely reduce the risk of prostate cancer. The recommended daily amount of fresh fruits and vegetables is about 4-5 cups. Most people have busy schedules and that is why I definitely believe that juicing is a great option. Although many kind of fruits and vegetables are extremely healthy, knowing which ones to combine to get the most benefit is the key. Green, red and orange fruits and vegetables are loaded with carotenoids which are especially beneficial for prostate cancer. Some of the best juice ingredients include: spinach, kale, dandelion greens, oranges, grapefruits, berries, carrots, and tomatoes. These tasty fruits and vegetables are the basis of juice recipes in this book. Most of these ingredients have a relatively neutral taste and can easily be combined with different herbs and spices for a superb taste.

These juices are powerful enough to boost up your immune system within a couple of days and help you prevent prostate cancer.

58 UNIQUE PROSTATE CANCER JUICE RECIPES: ALL-NATURAL HOME REMEDY SOLUTIONS THAT WILL GET YOUR BODY STRONGER AND HEALTHIER TO FIGHT CANCER CELLS

1.   Tomato Beet Juice

Ingredients:

4 cherry tomatoes, halved

2 whole beets, sliced

1 cup of watercress, torn

1 rosemary sprig

1 oz of water

Preparation:

Wash the tomatoes and remove the stems. Cut each in half and set aside.

Wash and trim off the beets. Cut the green parts and cut into thin slices. Set aside.

Place the watercress in a colander and wash under cold water. Torn with hands and set aside.

Now, combine tomatoes, beets, watercress, and rosemary in a juicer. Process until well juiced. Transfer to a serving glass and stir in the water. You can add some salt if you like, but it's optional.

Refrigerate for 10 minutes before serving.

Nutritional information per serving: Kcal: 63, Protein: 4.1g, Carbs: 18.7g, Fats: 0.4g

2.   Carrot Celery Juice

Ingredients:

1 large carrot, sliced

1 large celery, chopped

1 cup of fresh kale, chopped

1 small Granny Smith's apple, cored

1 tbsp of liquid honey

Preparation:

Wash and peel the carrot. Cut into thin slices and set aside.

Wash the celery and cut into bite-sized pieces. Set aside.

Rinse the kale under cold running water using a colander. Slightly drain and torn with hands. Set aside.

Wash the apple and cut lengthwise in half. Remove the core and cut into bite-sized pieces. Set aside.

Now, combine carrot, celery, kale, and apple in a juicer and process until juiced. Transfer to a serving glass and stir in the honey.

Add some ice and serve immediately.

Nutritional information per serving: Kcal: 179, Protein: 4.6g, Carbs: 34.3g, Fats: 1.1g

3.   Asparagus Grapefruit Juice

Ingredients:

1 cup of asparagus, trimmed and chopped

1 whole grapefruit, peeled

1 whole lime, peeled

1 whole leek, chopped

1 oz of water

Preparation:

Wash the asparagus and trim off the woody ends. Chop into small pieces and set aside.

Peel the grapefruit and divide into wedges. Cut each wedge in half and set aside.

Peel the lime and cut lengthwise in half. Set aside.

Wash the leek and cut into bite-sized pieces. Set aside.

Now, combine asparagus, grapefruit, lime, and leek in a juicer and process until well juiced. Transfer to a serving glass and stir in the water.

Add some honey if you like, but it's optional.

Refrigerate for 10 minutes before serving.

Enjoy!

Nutritional information per serving: Kcal: 161, Protein: 6.3g, Carbs: 47.7g, Fats: 0.8g

4.   Dandelion Juice

Ingredients:

1 cup of fresh dandelion greens, torn

2 medium-sized celery stalks, chopped

1 whole lemon, peeled

1 small Granny Smith's apple, cored

1 cup of cucumber, sliced

Preparation:

Wash dandelion greens thoroughly and torn with hands into small pieces. Set aside.

Wash the celery and cut into bite-sized pieces. Set aside.

Peel the lemon and cut lengthwise in half. Set aside.

Wash the apple and cut in half. Remove the core and cut into bite-sized pieces. Set aside.

Wash the cucumber and cut into thin slices. Fill the measuring cup and reserve the rest for later.

Now, combine dandelions, celery, lemon, apple, and cucumber in a juicer and process until juiced.

Transfer to a serving glass and add some crushed ice before serving.

Nutritional information per serving: Kcal: 97, Protein: 2.9g, Carbs: 29.7g, Fats: 0.7g

5. Broccoli Banana Juice

Ingredients:

1 cup of broccoli, chopped

1 large banana, sliced

1 small green apple, cored

1 small ginger knob, peeled

1 tbsp of liquid honey

Preparation:

Wash the broccoli and trim off the outer layers. Cut into small pieces and fill the measuring cup. Reserve the rest for later.

Peel the banana and cut into small slices. Set aside.

Wash the apple and cut in half. Remove the core and cut into bite-sized pieces. Set aside.

Peel the ginger knob and set aside.

Now, combine broccoli, banana, apple, and ginger in a juicer and process until well juiced. Transfer to a serving glass and stir in the honey.

Refrigerate for 10 minutes before serving.

Nutritional information per serving: Kcal: 261, Protein: 4.8g, Carbs: 57.7g, Fats: 1.1g

6.   Green Tea Juice

Ingredients:

1 tsp of green tea

2 tbsp of hot water

2 whole kiwis, peeled

1 medium-sized pear, chopped

1 cup of fresh spinach, torn

1 cup of fresh mint, roughly chopped

1 whole lime, peeled

Preparation:

Combine green tea and hot water in a small bowl. Stir well and set aside to soak for 3 minutes.

Peel the kiwis and cut lengthwise in half. Set aside.

Wash the pear and remove the core. Cut into bite-sized pieces and set aside.

Wash the spinach under cold running water using a colander. Torn with hands and set aside.

Wash the mint and roughly chop it. Fill the measuring cup and reserve the rest for later.

Peel the lime and cut lengthwise in half. Set aside.

Now, combine green tea mixture, kiwis, pear, spinach, mint, and lime in a juicer and process until juiced. Transfer to a serving glass and add some ice before serving.

Enjoy!

Nutritional information per serving: Kcal: 195, Protein: 9.4g, Carbs: 62.4g, Fats: 2.1g

7.   Pomegranate Asparagus Juice

Ingredients:

1 cup of pomegranate seeds

1 cup of fresh asparagus, trimmed and chopped

1 whole lemon, peeled

1 tbsp of liquid honey

1 oz of water

Preparation:

Cut the top of the pomegranate fruit using a sharp paring knife. Slice down to each of the white membranes inside of the fruit. Pop the seeds into a measuring cup and set aside.

Wash the asparagus and trim off the woody ends. Cut into bite-sized pieces and set aside.

Peel the lemon and cut into quarters. Set aside.

Now, combine pomegranate seeds, asparagus, and lemon in a juicer and process until well juiced. Transfer to a serving glass and stir in the honey and water.

Add some ice and enjoy!

Nutritional information per serving: Kcal: 145, Protein: 5.1g, Carbs: 26.8g, Fats: 1.3g

8.   Spinach Tomato Juice

Ingredients:

1 cup of fresh spinach, chopped

6 cherry tomatoes, halved

1 cup of cucumber, sliced

1 small ginger knob, peeled

¼ tsp of salt

Preparation:

Wash the spinach thoroughly under cold running water. Slightly drain and chop into small pieces. Set aside.

Wash the cherry tomatoes and remove the stems. Cut each tomato in half and set aside.

Wash the cucumber and cut into thin slices. Fill the measuring cup and reserve the rest for later.

Now, combine spinach, tomatoes, cucumber, and ginger in a juicer and process until juiced. Transfer to a serving glass and stir in the salt.

Serve immediately.

Nutritional information per serving: Kcal: 52, Protein: 7.4g, Carbs: 14.5g, Fats: 1.1g

9.   Watermelon Blueberry Juice

Ingredients:

1 cup of watermelon, cubed

2 cups of blueberries

1 whole lime, peeled

1 cup of fresh basil, torn

¼ tsp of cayenne pepper, ground

1 oz of water

Preparation:

Cut one large watermelon wedge. Using a sharp paring knife, peel and cut into small cubes. Remove the seeds and set aside.

Place the blueberries in a large colander. Rinse well under cold running water and set aside.

Peel the lime and cut lengthwise in half. Set aside.

Wash the basil and roughly torn it with hands. Set aside.

Now, combine watermelon, blueberries, lime, and basil in a juicer. Process until juiced. Transfer to a serving glass and stir in the cayenne pepper and water.

Refrigerate for 10 minutes before serving.

Nutritional information per serving: Kcal: 198, Protein: 4.1g, Carbs: 58.7g, Fats: 1.4g

10.   Carrot Plum Juice

Ingredients:

1 cup of baby carrots, sliced

4 whole plum, chopped

1 cup of Romaine lettuce, shredded

1 cup of mustard greens, torn

1 oz of water

Preparation:

Wash and peel the carrots. Cut into thin slices and fill the measuring cup. Reserve the rest in the refrigerator.

Wash the plums and cut each in half. Remove the pits and set aside.

Combine lettuce and mustard greens in a large colander. Rinse well under cold running water. Shred the lettuce torn the mustard greens using hands. Set aside.

Now, combine carrots, plums, lettuce, and mustard greens in a juicer and process until juiced. Transfer to a serving glass and stir in the water.

Serve cold.

Nutritional information per serving: Kcal: 128, Protein: 4.8g, Carbs: 39.1g, Fats: 1.3g

11. Pepper Avocado Juice

Ingredients:

2 medium-sized red bell peppers, chopped

1 cup of avocado, sliced

1 cup of purple cabbage, chopped

1 whole leek, chopped

1 whole lime, peeled

Preparation:

Wash the peppers and cut in half. Remove the seeds and cut into small pieces. Set aside.

Peel the avocado and cut lengthwise in half. Cut into thin slices and reserve the rest in the refrigerator. Set aside.

Wash the cabbage thoroughly and chop into small pieces. Set aside.

Wash the leek and cut into bite-sized pieces. Set aside.

Peel the lime and cut lengthwise in half. Set aside.

Now, combine peppers, avocado, cabbage, leek, and lime in a juicer and process until juiced. Transfer to a serving glass and refrigerate for 15 minutes before serving.

Enjoy!

Nutritional information per serving: Kcal: 327, Protein: 8.1g, Carbs: 49.6g, Fats: 22.5g

12. Grapefruit Mango Juice

Ingredients:

1 whole grapefruit, peeled

1 cup of mango, cut into chunks

1 cup of fresh mint, roughly chopped

1 large banana, peeled

2 large strawberries, chopped

Preparation:

Peel the grapefruit and divide into wedges. Cut each wedge in half and set aside.

Peel the mango and cut into small chunks. Fill the measuring cup and reserve the rest in the refrigerator. Set aside.

Wash the mint roughly and torn with hands. Set aside.

Peel the banana and cut into small pieces. Set aside.

Wash the strawberries and remove the stems. Cut into bite-sized pieces and set aside.

Now, combine grapefruit, mango, mint, banana, and strawberries in a juicer and process until juiced. Transfer to a serving glass and add some ice cubes before serving.

Enjoy!

Nutritional information per serving: Kcal: 301, Protein: 5.9g, Carbs: 88.5g, Fats: 1.7g

13.   Beet Lemon Juice

Ingredients:

1 whole beet, sliced

1 whole lemon, peeled

1 cup of cucumber, sliced

1 medium-sized orange, peeled

1 tbsp of liquid honey

Preparation:

Wash the beet and trim off the green parts. Cut into thin slices and set aside.

Peel the lemon and cut into quarters. Set aside.

Wash the cucumber and cut into thin slices. Fill the measuring cup and reserve the rest in the refrigerator.

Peel the orange and divide into wedges. Cut each wedge in half and set aside.

Now, combine beet, lemon, cucumber, and orange in a juicer and process until juiced. Transfer to a serving glass and stir in the honey.

Add some ice and serve immediately.

Nutritional information per serving: Kcal: 154, Protein: 3.5g, Carbs: 30.5g, Fats: 0.5g

14.   Green Bean Juice

Ingredients:

1 cup of green beans, chopped

1 medium-sized Granny Smith's apple, cored

1 medium-sized celery stalk, cut into bite-sized pieces

1 cup of fresh spinach, chopped

Preparation:

Wash the green beans and chop into bite-sized pieces. Fill the measuring cup and reserve the rest for later.

Wash the apple and cut in half. Remove the core and cut into small chunks. Set aside.

Wash the celery and cut into bite-sized pieces. Set aside.

Wash the spinach thoroughly under cold running water. Chop into small pieces and fill the measuring cup. Reserve the rest for later.

Now, combine green beans, apple, celery, and spinach in a juicer and process until well juiced. Transfer to serving glass and add some ice before serving.

Enjoy!

Nutritional information per serving: Kcal: 140, Protein: 8.5g, Carbs: 37.3g, Fats: 1.4g

15.   Pepper Kale Juice

Ingredients:

1 medium-sized red bell pepper, chopped

1 cup of fresh kale, chopped

1 cup of parsley, torn

1 large celery stalk, chopped

1 cup of cucumber, sliced

1 oz of water

Preparation:

Wash the bell pepper and cut lengthwise in half. Scrape out the seeds and remove the stem. Cut into bite-sized pieces and set aside.

Wash the kale thoroughly under cold running water. Slightly drain and chop it into small pieces. Set aside.

Wash the parsley and torn with hands. Fill the measuring cup and reserve the rest for later.

Wash the celery stalk and chop it into bite-sized pieces. Set aside.

Wash the cucumber and cut into thin slices. Fill the measuring cup and reserve the rest for later.

Now, combine bell pepper, kale, parsley, celery, and cucumber in a juicer and process until juiced. Transfer to a serving glass and stir in the water. Add some ice and serve immediately.

Enjoy!

Nutritional information per serving: Kcal: 77, Protein: 6.6g, Carbs: 20.6g, Fats: 1.6g

16.   Basil Zucchini Juice

Ingredients:

1 cup of fresh basil, chopped

1 medium-sized zucchini, sliced

1 whole lemon, peeled

1 whole lime, peeled

1 oz of water

Preparation:

Wash the basil thoroughly under cold running water. Slightly drain and chop into small pieces. Set aside.

Wash the zucchini and cut into thin slices. Set aside.

Peel the lemon and lime. Cut each fruit into quarters and set aside.

Now, combine basil, zucchini, lemon, and lime in a juicer. Process until well juiced. Transfer to a serving glass and stir in the water.

Refrigerate for 10 minutes before serving.

Nutritional information per serving: Kcal: 50, Protein: 3.9g, Carbs: 15.8g, Fats: 0.9g

17. Blueberry Grape Juice

Ingredients:

1 cup of blueberries

1 cup of black grapes

1 small Golden Delicious apple, cored

¼ tsp of cinnamon, ground

Preparation:

Wash the blueberries using a colander. Slightly drain and set aside.

Wash the grapes and fill the measuring cup. Reserve the rest for later.

Wash the apple and cut in half. Remove the core and cut into bite-sized pieces. Set aside.

Now, combine blueberries, grapes, and apple in a juicer and process until juiced. Transfer to a serving glass and stir in the cinnamon.

Add some ice before serving and enjoy!

Nutritional information per serving: Kcal: 191, Protein: 2.1g, Carbs: 54.7g, Fats: 1g

18.   Mango Raspberry Juice

Ingredients:

1 cup of mango, chunked

1 cup of raspberries

1 small peach, pitted

3 whole apricots, chopped

Preparation:

Peel the mango and cut into small chunks. Fill the measuring cup and reserve the rest for later.

Wash the raspberries using a colander. Slightly drain and fill the measuring cup. Reserve the rest in the refrigerator or freezer for later.

Wash the peach and cut in half. Remove the pit and cut into bite-sized pieces. Set aside.

Wash the apricots and cut in half. Remove the pits and cut in quarters. Set aside.

Now, combine mango, raspberries, peach, and apricots in a juicer and process until juiced. Transfer to a serving glass refrigerate for 10 minutes before serving.

You can garnish with some fresh mint if you like, but it's optional.

Nutritional information per serving: Kcal: 206, Protein: 5.5g, Carbs: 63.5g, Fats: 2.1g

19.   Pineapple Beet Juice

Ingredients:

1 cup of pineapple, chunked

1 whole beet, sliced

1 small orange, wedged

2 tbsp of coconut water

¼ tsp of ginger, ground

Preparation:

Cut the top of a pineapple and peel it using a sharp paring knife. Cut into small chunks and fill the measuring cup. Reserve the rest of the pineapple in a refrigerator.

Wash and trim off the beet. Cut into small slices and set aside.

Peel the orange and divide into wedges. Cut each wedge in half and set aside.

Now, combine pineapple, beet, and orange in a juicer and process until juiced. Transfer to a serving glass and stir in the coconut water and ginger.

Add some crushed ice and serve immediately.

Nutritional information per serving: Kcal: 135, Protein: 3.1g, Carbs: 40.7g, Fats: 0.5g

20. Kiwi Banana Juice

Ingredients:

3 whole kiwis, peeled

1 large banana, chopped

1 large strawberry, chopped

1 small apple, cored

¼ tsp of cinnamon, ground

Preparation:

Peel the kiwis and cut lengthwise in half. Set aside.

Peel the banana and chop into small chunks. Set aside.

Wash the strawberry and remove the stem. Cut into small pieces and set aside.

Wash the apple and cut in half. Remove the core and cut into bite-sized pieces. Set aside.

Now, combine kiwis, banana, strawberry, and apple in a juicer and process until juiced. Transfer to a serving glass and stir in the cinnamon.

Refrigerate for 10 minutes before serving.

Enjoy!

Nutritional information per serving: Kcal: 292, Protein: 4.4g, Carbs: 85g, Fats: 1.9g

21.   Avocado Lemon Juice

Ingredients:

1 cup of avocado, cubed

1 whole lemon, peeled

1 cup of cranberries

1 cup of cucumber, sliced

1 cup of cherries, pitted

Preparation:

Peel the avocado and cut into small cubes. Fill the measuring cup and reserve the rest in the refrigerator. Set aside.

Peel the lemon and cut lengthwise in half. Set aside.

Wash the cranberries and set aside.

Wash the cucumber and cut into slices. Fill the measuring cup and reserve the the rest for later.

Wash the cherries and cut each in half. Remove the pits and set aside.

Now, combine avocado, cranberries, cucumber, and cherries in a juicer and process until juiced. Transfer to a serving glass and add some ice before serving.

Enjoy!

Nutritional information per serving: Kcal: 321, Protein: 5.8g, Carbs: 54.4g, Fats: 22.6g

22.   Pomegranate Blackberry Juice

Ingredients:

1 cup of pomegranate seeds

1 cup of blackberries

1 whole lemon, peeled

1 medium-sized carrot, sliced

1 oz of water

Preparation:

Cut the top of the pomegranate fruit using a sharp paring knife. Slice down to each of the white membranes inside of the fruit. Pop the seeds into a measuring cup and set aside.

Wash the blackberries using a colander. Fill the measuring cup and reserve the rest. Set aside.

Peel the lemon and cut lengthwise in half. Set aside.

Wash and peel the carrot. Cut into thin slices and set aside.

Now, combine pomegranate seeds, blackberries, lemon, and carrot in a juicer. Process until juiced and transfer to a serving glass.

Add some ice or refrigerate for a while before serving.

Nutritional information per serving: Kcal: 119, Protein: 4.6g, Carbs: 41.3g, Fats: 2.1g

23.   Celery Kale Juice

Ingredients:

1 cup of celery, chopped

1 cup of fresh kale, torn

1 cup of fresh mint, torn

1 whole lime, peeled

1 small Granny Smith's apple, cored

Preparation:

Wash the celery and chop into small pieces. Fill the measuring cup and set aside.

Combine kale and mint in a large colander. Wash thoroughly under cold running water. Slightly drain and torn with hands. Set aside.

Peel the lime and cut into small pieces. Set aside.

Wash the apple and cut in half. Remove the core and cut into bite-sized pieces. Set aside.

Now, combine celery, kale, mint, lime, and apple in a juicer and process until juiced. Transfer to a serving glass and add some ice before serving.

Enjoy!

Nutritional information per serving: Kcal: 121, Protein: 5.3g, Carbs: 35.8g, Fats: 1.3g

24.   Potato Zucchini Juice

Ingredients:

1 cup of sweet potatoes, cubed

1 small zucchini, sliced

1 small apple, cored

¼ tsp of ginger, ground

Preparation:

Peel the sweet potato and cut into small cubes. Fill the measuring cup and reserve the rest for later.

Peel the zucchini and cut into thin slices. Set aside.

Wash the apple and cut in half. Remove the core and cut into bite-sized pieces. Set aside.

Now, combine sweet potatoes, zucchini, and apple in a juicer. Process until well juiced. Transfer to a serving glass and stir in the ginger.

Refrigerate for 10 minutes before serving.

Enjoy!

Nutritional information per serving: Kcal: 181, Protein: 4.2g, Carbs: 50.1g, Fats: 0.7g

25.   Apricot Plum Juice

Ingredients:

2 whole apricots, pitted

2 whole plums, chopped

1 cup of cherries, pitted

1 small orange, peeled

1 tbsp of coconut water

Preparation:

Wash the apricots and cut in half. Remove the pits and cut all into small pieces. Set aside.

Wash the plums and cut in half. Remove the pits and cut into bite-sized pieces. Set aside.

Wash the cherries using a colander. Remove the pits and set aside.

Peel the orange and divide into wedges. Cut each wedge in half and set aside.

Now, combine apricots, plums, cherries, and orange in a juicer and process until well juiced. Transfer to a serving glass and stir in the coconut water.

Refrigerate for 10 minutes before serving.

Enjoy!

Nutritional information per serving: Kcal: 191, Protein: 4.3g, Carbs: 56.3g, Fats: 1.1g

26.   Fennel Broccoli Juice

Ingredients:

1 cup of fennel, chopped

1 cup of broccoli, chopped

1 cup of Brussels sprouts, halved

1 cup of watercress, torn

1 cup of cucumber, sliced

Preparation:

Wash the fennel and trim off the outer leaves. Using a sharp paring knife, cut into small pieces and fill the measuring cup. Reserve the rest for later.

Wash the broccoli and cut into small pieces. Fill the measuring cup and reserve the rest in the refrigerator. Set aside.

Wash the Brussels sprouts and trim off the outer layers. Cut in half and set aside.

Wash the watercress thoroughly under cold running water. Slightly drain and torn with hands. Set aside.

Wash the cucumber and cut into thin slices. Fill the measuring cup and reserve the rest for later.

Now, combine fennel, broccoli, Brussels sprouts, watercress, and cucumber in a juicer and process until juiced. Transfer to a serving glass and refrigerate for 10 minutes before serving.

Enjoy!

Nutritional information per serving: Kcal: 72, Protein: 7.7g, Carbs: 22.6g, Fats: 0.8g

27. Cranberry Pear Juice

Ingredients:

1 cup of cranberries

1 medium-sized pear, chopped

1 whole lemon, peeled

½ cup of strawberries, sliced

1 small ginger knob, peeled

1 oz of water

Preparation:

Wash the cranberries and fill the measuring cup. Set aside.

Wash the pear and cut in half. Remove the core and cut into small pieces. Set aside.

Peel the lemon and cut in half. Set aside.

Wash the strawberries and remove the stems. Cut into small pieces and fill the measuring cup. Set aside.

Peel the ginger knob and set aside.

Now, combine cranberries, pear, lemon, strawberries, and ginger in a juicer and process until juiced. Transfer to a serving glass and stir in the water.

Serve cold.

Nutritional information per serving: Kcal: 143, Protein: 2.4g, Carbs: 52.7g, Fats: 0.8g

28.   Beet Green Carrot Juice

Ingredients:

1 cup of beet greens, torn

1 large carrot, sliced

1 medium-sized orange, peeled

1 cup of cantaloupe, chopped

¼ tsp of ginger, ground

Preparation:

Wash the beet greens thoroughly under cold running water. Drain and torn with hands. Set aside.

Wash the carrot and cut into thin slices. Set aside.

Peel the orange and divide into wedges. Cut each wedge in half and set aside.

Cut the cantaloupe in half. Scoop out the seeds and cut one large wedge. Peel it and cut into small pieces. Fill the measuring cup and reserve the rest of the cantaloupe in a refrigerator.

Now, combine beet greens, carrot, orange, and cantaloupe in a juicer and process until juiced. Transfer to a serving glass and stir in the ginger.

Serve cold.

Nutritional information per serving: Kcal: 99, Protein: 3.5g, Carbs: 30.5g, Fats: 0.6g

29.   Collard Greens Cucumber Juice

Ingredients:

2 cups of collard greens, chopped

1 cup of cucumber, sliced

1 whole lime, peeled

1 cup of Swiss chard, chopped

1 large celery stalk, chopped

1 oz of water

¼ tsp of salt

Preparation:

Combine collard greens and Swiss chard in a large colander. Wash it under running water and slightly drain. Chop into small pieces and set aside.

Wash the cucumber and cut into thin slices. Fill the measuring cup and reserve the rest in the refrigerator.

Peel the lime and cut lengthwise in half. Set aside.

Wash the celery and cut into small pieces. Set aside.

Now, combine collard greens, cucumber, lime, Swiss chard, and celery in a juicer and process until juiced. Transfer to a serving glass and stir in the water and salt. Refrigerate for 10 minutes before serving.

Enjoy!

Nutritional information per serving: Kcal: 40, Protein: 3.8g, Carbs: 12.7g, Fats: 0.7g

30.   Pumpkin Pepper Juice

Ingredients:

1 cup of pumpkin, cubed

1 large yellow bell pepper, chopped

1 small zucchini, sliced

¼ tsp of cinnamon, ground

Preparation:

Cut the pumpkin lengthwise in half. Scoop out the seeds and cut one large wedge. Peel it and fill the measuring cup. Wrap the rest of the pumpkin in a plastic foil and refrigerate for later.

Wash the bell pepper and cut in half. Remove the seeds and stem. Cut into bite-sized pieces and set aside.

Wash the zucchini thoroughly and cut into thin slices. Set aside.

Now, combine pumpkin, bell pepper, and zucchini in a juicer and process until juiced. Transfer to a serving glass and stir in the cinnamon.

Refrigerate for 10 minutes before serving.

Enjoy!

Nutritional information per serving: Kcal: 86, Protein: 4.5g, Carbs: 22.9g, Fats: 0.9g

31.   Kale Celery Juice

Ingredients:

1 cup of fresh kale, chopped

2 medium-sized celery stalk, chopped

1 small apple, cored

1 cup of Romaine lettuce, shredded

Preparation:

Wash the kale thoroughly under cold running water. Slightly drain and chop it into small pieces. Set aside.

Wash the celery stalks and cut into bite-sized pieces. Set aside.

Wash the apple and cut in half. remove the core and cut into small pieces. Set aside.

Wash the lettuce leaves and shred it. Fill the measuring cup and reserve the rest for later.

Now, combine kale, celery, apple, and lettuce in a juicer and process until juiced. Transfer to a serving glass and add some ice before serving.

Enjoy!

Nutritional information per serving: Kcal: 103, Protein: 4.6g, Carbs: 29.4g, Fats: 1.2g

32.   Melon Lime Juice

Ingredients:

1 medium-sized wedge of honeydew melon

1 whole lime, peeled

1 small Granny Smith's apple, cored

1 large banana, peeled

¼ tsp of cinnamon, ground

Preparation:

Cut one large honeydew melon wedge and peel it. Remove the seeds and cut into bite-sized pieces. Wrap the rest of the melon in a plastic foil and refrigerate.

Peel the lime and cut lengthwise in half. Set aside.

Wash the apple and cut in half. Remove the core and cut into bite-sized pieces. Set aside.

Peel the banana and chop into small chunks. Set aside.

Now, combine melon, lime, apple, and banana in a juicer and process until juiced. Transfer to a serving glass and stir in the cinnamon.

Refrigerate for 10 minutes before serving.

Nutritional information per serving: Kcal: 226, Protein: 4.6g, Carbs: 29.4g, Fats: 1.2g

33. Guava Cherry Juice

Ingredients:

1 whole guava, peeled

1 cup of cherries, pitted

1 medium-sized orange, wedged

1 whole apricot, pitted

Preparation:

Peel the guava and cut into small chunks. Set aside.

Wash the cherries using a colander. Remove the stems and cut each in half. Remove the pits and fill the measuring cup. Set aside.

Peel the orange and divide into wedges. Cut each wedge in half and set aside.

Wash the apricot and cut in half. Remove the pit and cut into bite-sized pieces. Set aside.

Now, combine guava, cherries, orange, and apricot in a juicer and process until juiced. Transfer to a serving glass and add some ice.

Serve immediately.

Nutritional information per serving: Kcal: 173, Protein: 4.7g, Carbs: 51.8g, Fats: 1.1g

34.   Mango Kiwi Juice

Ingredients:

1 cup of mango, chunked

1 whole kiwi, peeled

1 cup of fresh spinach, chopped

1 small ginger knob, peeled

2 tbsp of coconut water

Preparation:

Peel the mango and cut into small chunks. Fill the measuring cup and reserve the rest in the refrigerator.

Peel the kiwi and cut lengthwise in half. Set aside.

Wash the spinach thoroughly under cold running water. Slightly drain and chop it into small pieces. Set aside.

Peel the ginger knob and set aside.

Now, combine mango, kiwi, spinach, and ginger in a juicer and process until juiced. Transfer to a serving glass and stir in the coconut water. Refrigerate for 10 minutes before serving.

Enjoy!

Nutritional information per serving: Kcal: 190, Protein: 9.1g, Carbs: 53.6g, Fats: 2.2g

35.   Pomegranate Plum Juice

Ingredients:

1 cup of pomegranate seeds

2 whole plums, pitted

1 small Golden Delicious apple, cored

1 large strawberry, chopped

Preparation:

Cut the top of the pomegranate fruit using a sharp paring knife. Slice down to each of the white membranes inside of the fruit. Pop the seeds into a measuring cup and set aside.

Wash the plums and cut lengthwise in half. Remove the pits and cut into small pieces. Set aside.

Wash the apple and cut in half. Remove the core and cut into bite-sized pieces. Set aside.

Wash the strawberry and remove the stem. Cut into small pieces and set aside.

Now, combine pomegranate seeds, plums, apple, and strawberry in a juicer and process until juiced. Transfer to a serving glass and add some crushed ice.

Serve immediately.

Nutritional information per serving: Kcal: 176, Protein: 2.8g, Carbs: 50.3g, Fats: 1.6g

36.   Watermelon Cranberry Juice

Ingredients:

1 cup of watermelon, chopped

1 cup of whole cranberries

1 whole lemon, peeled

1 cup of fresh mint, chopped

1 tbsp of liquid honey

Preparation:

Cut the watermelon lengthwise. For one cup, you will need a large slice. Peel and cut into chunks. Remove the seeds and set aside. Reserve the rest for some other juices.

Wash the cranberries using a colander. Fill the measuring cup and reserve the rest in the refrigerator.

Peel the lemon and cut lengthwise in half. Set aside.

Wash the mint thoroughly under cold running water and roughly chop it. Set aside.

Now, combine watermelon, cranberries, lemon, and mint in a juicer and process until juiced. Transfer to a serving glass and stir in the honey.

Add few ice cubes and serve immediately.

Enjoy!

Nutritional information per serving: Kcal: 93, Protein: 2.9g, Carbs: 32.8g, Fats: 0.7g

37. Grape Pineapple Juice

Ingredients:

1 cup of black grapes

1 cup of pineapple, chunked

1 tsp of vanilla extract

Preparation:

In a heavy-bottomed pot, combine grapes and one cup of water. Bring it to a boil over a medium-high temperature, stirring occasionally. Stir in the vanilla extract and remove from the heat. Set aside to cool completely.

Cut the top of a pineapple fruit. Using a sharp paring knife, peel it and cut into thin slices. Fill the measuring cup and reserve the rest for later.

Now, combine grape mixture and pineapple in a juicer and process until well juiced. Transfer to a serving glass and refrigerate for 20 minutes before serving.

Garnish with some fresh mint, but it's optional.

Enjoy!

Nutritional information per serving: Kcal: 200, Protein: 2.1g, Carbs: 57g, Fats: 0.8g

38.   Tomato Celery Juice

Ingredients:

5 cherry tomatoes, halved

1 large celery stalk, chopped

1 cup of cucumber, sliced

1 cup of fresh parsley, chopped

¼ tsp of salt

¼ tsp of black pepper, ground

½ tsp of Tabasco sauce

1 oz of water

Preparation:

Wash the cherry tomatoes and remove the stems. Cut each tomato in half and set aside.

Wash the celery stalk and chop it into bite-sized pieces. Set aside.

Wash the cucumber and cut into thin slices. Fill the measuring cup and reserve the rest for later.

Place the parsley in a colander and rinse it thoroughly. Slightly drain and chop into small pieces. Set aside.

Now, combine cherry tomatoes, celery, cucumber, and parsley in a juicer and process until juiced. Transfer to a serving glass and stir in the salt, pepper, Tabasco sauce, and water.

Serve immediately!

Nutritional information per serving: Kcal: 38, Protein: 3.3g, Carbs: 10.9g, Fats: 0.8g

39.   Blueberry Ginger Juice

Ingredients:

2 cups of blueberries

1 small ginger knob, peeled and chopped

1 medium-sized blood orange, peeled

1 cup of black grapes

Preparation:

Place the blueberries in a colander. Wash thoroughly under cold running water and drain. Fill the measuring cups and reserve the rest in the freezer.

Peel the ginger and cut into small pieces. Set aside.

Peel the orange and divide into wedges. Cut each wedge in half and set aside.

Wash the grapes and fill the measuring cup. Set aside.

Now, combine blueberries, ginger, orange, and grapes in a juicer and process until juiced. Transfer to a serving glass and add few ice cubes before serving.

Enjoy!

Nutritional information per serving: Kcal: 254, Protein: 4.1g, Carbs: 75.2g, Fats: 1.5g

40.   Avocado Papaya Juice

Ingredients:

1 cup of avocado, cubed

1 small papaya, chopped

1 cup of cherries, halved

1 whole lemon, peeled

¼ tsp of cinnamon, ground

1 oz of water

Preparation:

Peel the avocado and cut lengthwise in half. Remove the pit and cut into small cubes. Fill the measuring cup and reserve the rest for later.

Peel the papaya and cut into small chunks. Set aside.

Peel the lemon and cut lengthwise in half. Set aside.

Now, combine avocado, papaya, and lemon in a juicer and process until juiced. Transfer to a serving glass and stir in the cinnamon and water.

Refrigerate for 15 minutes before serving and enjoy!

Nutritional information per serving: Kcal: 343, Protein: 5.8g, Carbs: 57.3g, Fats: 22.8g

41.   Pumpkin Apple Juice

Ingredients:

1 cup of pumpkin, cubed

1 small Granny Smith's apple, cored

1 medium-sized carrot, sliced

1 cup of cucumber, sliced

¼ tsp of cinnamon, ground

¼ tsp of ginger, ground

Preparation:

Cut the pumpkin in half and scoop out the seeds. Wash it and cut one large wedge. Peel it and cut into small cubes. Fill the measuring cup and reserve the rest in the refrigerator.

Wash the apple and cut lengthwise in half. Remove the core and cut into small pieces. Set aside.

Wash and peel the carrot. Cut into thin slices and set aside.

Wash the cucumber and cut into thin slices. Fill the measuring cup and reserve the rest for later.

Now, combine pumpkin, apple, carrot, and cucumber in a juicer and process until juiced. Transfer to a serving glass and stir in the cinnamon and ginger.

Refrigerate for 10 minutes before serving.

Nutritional information per serving: Kcal: 121, Protein: 2.7g, Carbs: 34.8g, Fats: 0.6g

42.   Peach Lime Juice

Ingredients:

2 large peaches, pitted

1 whole lime, peeled

1 cup of apricots, sliced

1 large banana, peeled

Preparation:

Wash the peaches and cut in half. Remove the pits and cut each half into bite-sized pieces. Set aside.

Peel the lime and roughly chop it. Make sure to reserve lime juice while cutting.

Wash the apricots and cut in half. Remove the pits and cut into small pieces. Fill the measuring cup and set aside.

Peel the banana and cut into small chunks. Set aside.

Now, combine peaches, lime, apricots, and banana in a juicer and process until juiced. Transfer to a serving glass and add some crushed ice before serving.

Enjoy!

Nutritional information per serving: Kcal: 299, Protein: 7.2g, Carbs: 86.5g, Fats: 2g

43.   Artichoke Spinach Juice

Ingredients:

1 medium-sized artichoke, chopped

1 cup of fresh spinach, chopped

1 cup of green beans, chopped

1 small green bell pepper, sliced

1 small ginger knob, peeled and sliced

Preparation:

Trim off the outer leaves of the artichoke using a sharp paring knife. Wash it and cut into bite-sized pieces. Set aside.

Using a colander, rinse the spinach thoroughly under cold running water. Chop into small pieces and set aside.

Place the beans in a deep pot. Add 1 cup of water and bring it to a boil. Cook for 5 minutes and remove from the heat. Set aside to cool completely.

Wash the bell pepper and cut in half. Remove the seeds and stem. Cut into small rings and set aside.

Peel the ginger knob and chop it into small pieces. Set aside.

Now, combine artichoke, spinach, green beans, bell pepper, and ginger in a juicer and process until juiced. Transfer to a serving glass and refrigerate for 10 minutes before serving.

Nutritional information per serving: Kcal: 95, Protein: 11.9g, Carbs: 29.4g, Fats: 1.3g

44.   Orange Pear Juice

Ingredients:

1 medium-sized orange, peeled

1 medium-sized pear, chopped

1 whole plum, pitted

1 whole lemon, peeled

1 oz of water

Preparation:

Peel the orange and divide into wedges. Cut each wedge in half and set aside.

Wash the pear and cut in half. Remove the core and chop into small pieces. Set aside.

Wash the plum and cut in half. Remove the pit and cut in small pieces.

Peel the lemon and cut into quarters. Set aside.

Now, combine orange, pear, plum, and lemon in a juicer and process until juiced. Transfer to a serving glass and stir in the water.

You can add a pinch of minced mint for some extra smooth flavor, but it's optional.

Add some crushed ice and serve immediately.

Nutritional information per serving: Kcal: 166, Protein: 2.9g, Carbs: 55.4g, Fats: 0.8g

45. Carrot Grapefruit Juice

Ingredients:

2 medium-sized carrots, sliced

1 whole grapefruit, wedged

1 cup of Romaine lettuce, shredded

1 cup of fresh mint, chopped

1 whole lime, peeled

Preparation:

Wash and peel the carrots. Cut into thin slices and set aside.

Peel the grapefruit and divide into wedges. Cut each wedge in half and set aside.

Wash the lettuce thoroughly under cold running water. Shred it and fill the measuring cup. Reserve the rest for later.

Wash the mint and then place it in a medium bowl. Add one cup of hot water and let it soak for 10 minutes. Slightly drain and set aside.

Peel the lime and cut lengthwise in half. Set aside.

Now, combine carrots, grapefruit, lettuce, mint, and lime in a juicer and process until juiced. Transfer to a serving glass and add some crushed ice before serving.

Enjoy!

Nutritional information per serving: Kcal: 147, Protein: 4.7g, Carbs: 46.8g, Fats: 1.1g

46.   Swiss Chard Juice

Ingredients:

2 cups of Swiss chard, chopped

1 cup of fresh kale, chopped

1 cup of collard greens, chopped

1 whole lemon, peeled

1 cup of cucumber, sliced

¼ tsp of ginger, ground

Preparation:

Combine Swiss chard, kale, and collard greens in a large colander. Wash thoroughly under cold running water. Slightly drain and roughly chop all. Set aside.

Peel the lemon and cut lengthwise in half. Set aside.

Wash the cucumber and cut into thin slices. Fill the measuring cup and reserve the rest in the refrigerator. Set aside.

Now, combine Swiss chard, kale, collard greens, lemon, and cucumber in a juicer. Process until juiced.

Transfer to a serving glass and stir in the ginger.

Serve cold.

Nutritional information per serving: Kcal: 57, Protein: 6.3g, Carbs: 17.8g, Fats: 1.2g

47.   Broccoli Brussels Sprout Juice

Ingredients:

1 cup of broccoli, chopped

1 cup of Brussels sprouts, halved

1 cup of cucumber, sliced

1 whole lime, peeled

¼ tsp of ginger, ground

Preparation:

Wash the broccoli and trim off the outer layers. Cut into small pieces and fill the measuring cup. Set aside.

Wash the Brussels sprouts and trim off the outer leaves. Cut each sprout in half and fill the measuring cup. Reserve the rest for in the refrigerator.

Wash the cucumber and cut into thin slices. Fill the measuring cup and reserve the rest for later. Set aside.

Peel the lime and cut lengthwise in half.

Now, combine broccoli, Brussels sprouts, cucumber, and lime in a juicer and process until juiced. Transfer to a serving glass and stir in the ginger.

Add few ice cubes and serve immediately.

Nutritional information per serving: Kcal: 63, Protein: 6.1g, Carbs: 19.5g, Fats: 1.2g

48.   Blackberry Avocado Juice

Ingredients:

2 cups of blackberries

1 cup of avocado, cubed

1 medium-sized apple, cored

¼ tsp of ginger, ground

Preparation:

Place the blackberries in a colander and wash thoroughly under cold running water. Slightly drain and set aside.

Peel the avocado and cut lengthwise in half. Remove the pit and cut into small cubes. Fill the measuring cup and reserve the rest in the refrigerator.

Wash the apple and cut in half. Remove the core and cut into bite-sized pieces. Set aside.

Now, combine blackberries, avocado, and apple in a juicer and process until juiced. Transfer to a serving glass and stir in the ginger.

Add some ice and serve immediately.

Nutritional information per serving: Kcal: 342, Protein: 7.7g, Carbs: 63.2g, Fats: 23.7g

49.   Raspberry Pear Juice

Ingredients:

1 cup of raspberries

1 large pear, chopped

1 whole lemon, peeled

1 small green apple, cored

Preparation:

Wash the raspberries thoroughly using a colander. Slightly drain and set aside.

Wash the pear and cut in half. Remove the core and cut into bite-sized pieces. Set aside.

Peel the lemon and cut lengthwise in half. Set aside.

Wash the apple and cut in half. Remove the core and cut into small pieces. Set aside.

Now, combine raspberries, pear, lemon, and apple in a juicer and process until juiced. Transfer to a serving glass and add some ice before serving.

Enjoy!

Nutritional information per serving: Kcal: 214, Protein: 3.6g, Carbs: 74.7g, Fats: 1.6g

50.   Coco Squash Juice

Ingredients:

1 cup of crookneck squash, sliced

1 medium-sized pear, chopped

1 cup of cucumber, sliced

1 whole lime, peeled

1 oz of coconut water

Preparation:

Peel the crookneck squash and scrape out the seeds with a spoon. Cut into small cubes and fill the measuring cup. Reserve the rest of the squash for some other recipe. Wrap in a plastic foil and refrigerate.

Wash the pear and cut in half. Remove the core and chop into small pieces. Set aside.

Wash the cucumber and cut into thin slices. Fill the measuring cup and reserve the rest in the refrigerator. Set aside.

Peel the lime and cut lengthwise in half. Set aside.

Now, combine squash, pear, cucumber, and lime in a juicer. Process until juiced. Transfer to a serving glass and stir in the coconut water.

Add some ice and serve immediately.

Nutritional information per serving: Kcal: 120, Protein: 2.4g, Carbs: 37.6g, Fats: 0.7g

51.   Kiwi Papaya Juice

Ingredients:

4 whole kiwis, peeled

2 small papaya, chopped

1 tbsp of fresh basil, roughly chopped

1 large banana, peeled

1 cup of cucumber, sliced

Preparation:

Peel the kiwis and cut in half. Set aside.

Peel the papaya and cut in half. Remove the seeds and dice into small pieces. Set aside.

Peel the banana and cut into chunks. Set aside.

Wash the cucumber and cut into thin slices. Fill the measuring cup and reserve the rest for later. Set aside.

Now, combine kiwis, papaya, basil, banana, and cucumber in a juicer and process until juiced. Transfer to a serving glass and add some ice before serving.

Enjoy!

Nutritional information per serving: Kcal: 365, Protein: 6.5g, Carbs: 107g, Fats: 2.8g

52.   Pepper Broccoli Juice

Ingredients:

1 large red bell pepper, chopped

1 cup of broccoli, chopped

1 cup of cucumber, sliced

1 large celery stalk, chopped

¼ tsp of ginger, ground

Preparation:

Wash the pepper and cut in half. Remove the seeds and stem. Cut into thin slices and set aside.

Wash the broccoli and trim off the outer wilted layers. Cut into small pieces and set aside.

Wash the cucumber and cut into thin slices. Fill the measuring cup and reserve the rest in the refrigerator.

Wash the celery stalk and cut into small pieces. Set aside.

Now, combine pepper, broccoli, cucumber, and celery in a juicer and process until well juiced. Transfer to a serving glass and stir in the ginger.

Refrigerate for 10 minutes before serving.

Nutritional information per serving: Kcal: 71, Protein: 4.9g, Carbs: 19.7g, Fats: 1g

53. Cantaloupe Orange Juice

Ingredients:

1 cup of cantaloupe, diced

1 small orange, peeled

1 cup of fresh mint, torn

1 whole lemon, peeled

¼ tsp of ginger, ground

Preparation:

Cut the cantaloupe in half. Scoop out the seeds and cut one medium wedge. Peel it and dice into small pieces. Reserve the rest of the cantaloupe in a refrigerator.

Peel the orange and divide into wedges. Cut each wedge in half and set aside.

Wash the mint thoroughly under cold water. Slightly drain and torn with hands. Set aside.

Peel the lemon and cut lengthwise in half. Set aside.

Now, combine cantaloupe, orange, mint, and lemon in a juicer and process until juiced. Transfer to a serving glass and stir in the ginger.

Add some ice before serving and enjoy!

Nutritional information per serving: Kcal: 104, Protein: 3.8g, Carbs: 33.2g, Fats: 0.8g

54. Tomato Greens Juice

Ingredients:

7 cherry tomatoes, halved

2 cups of Swiss chard, torn

2 cups of collard greens, torn

1 cup of cucumber, sliced

1 whole leek, chopped

Preparation:

Wash the tomatoes and remove the stems. Cut each tomato in half and set aside.

Combine Swiss chard and collard greens in a large colander. Wash thoroughly under cold running water. Slightly drain and torn with hands. Set aside.

Wash the cucumber and cut into thin slices. Fill the measuring cup and reserve the rest for later.

Wash the leek and cut into small pieces. Set aside.

Now, combine tomatoes, Swiss chard, collard greens, cucumber, and leek in a juicer and process until juiced.

Transfer to a serving glass and refrigerate for 10 minutes before serving.

Nutritional information per serving: Kcal: 91, Protein: 6.2g, Carbs: 25.7g, Fats: 1.1g

55.   Mango Citrus Juice

Ingredients:

1 cup of mango, chunked

1 whole lemon, peeled

1 whole lime, peeled

1 small green apple, cored

1 tbsp of coconut water

¼ tsp of cinnamon, ground

Preparation:

Peel the mango and cut into small chunks. Fill the measuring cup and reserve the rest for later.

Peel the lemon and lime. Cut each fruit in half and set aside.

Wash the apple and cut in half. Remove the core and cut into bite-sized pieces. Set aside.

Now, combine mango, lemon, lime, and apple in a juicer and process until juiced. Transfer to a serving glass and stir in the coconut water and cinnamon.

Add some crushed ice and serve immediately.

Nutritional information per serving: Kcal: 178, Protein: 2.8g, Carbs: 53.4g, Fats: 1.1g

56. Beet Kale Juice

Ingredients:

1 whole beet, sliced

1 cup of fresh kale, torn

1 small green apple, cored

1 small orange, peeled

¼ tsp of ginger, ground

Preparation:

Wash and trim off the beet. Slightly peel and cut into thin slices. Set aside.

Place the kale in a colander and wash under running water. Drain and torn with hands. Set aside.

Wash the apple and cut in half. Remove the core and cut into bite-sized pieces. Set aside.

Peel the orange and divide into wedges. Cut each wedge in half and set aside.

Now, combine beet, kale, apple, and orange in a juicer and process until juiced. Transfer to a serving glass and stir in the ginger.

Add some crushed ice and serve immediately.

Nutritional information per serving: Kcal: 153, Protein: 5.7g, Carbs: 44.6g, Fats: 1.1g

57. Blueberry Kiwi Juice

Ingredients:

1 cup of blueberries

2 whole kiwis, peeled

1 whole lemon, peeled

1 cup of cantaloupe, diced

1 tbsp of coconut water

Preparation:

Place the blueberries in a colander. Wash thoroughly and drain. Set aside.

Peel the kiwis and lemon. Cut lengthwise in half and set aside.

Cut the cantaloupe in half. Scoop out the seeds and cut one large wedge. Peel it and cut into small pieces. Fill the measuring cup and reserve the rest of the cantaloupe in a refrigerator.

Now, combine blueberries, kiwis, lemon, and cantaloupe in a juicer and process until juiced. Transfer to a serving glass and stir in the coconut water.

Refrigerate for 10 minutes before serving.

Nutritional information per serving: Kcal: 196, Protein: 4.6g, Carbs: 59.8g, Fats: 1.6g

58. Cauliflower Spinach Juice

Ingredients:

5 cauliflower flowerets, chopped

1 cup of fresh spinach, torn

1 cup of pomegranate seeds

1 oz of water

¼ tsp of ginger, ground

Preparation:

Wash the cauliflower flowerets and chop into small pieces. Fill the measuring cup and reserve the rest for later.

Wash the spinach thoroughly under running water. Torn with hands and set aside.

Cut the top of the pomegranate fruit using a sharp paring knife. Slice down to each of the white membranes inside of the fruit. Pop the seeds into a measuring cup and set aside.

Now, combine cauliflower, spinach, and pomegranate in a juicer and process until juiced. Transfer to a serving glass and stir in the water and ginger.

Add some ice and serve immediately.

Nutritional information per serving: Kcal: 162, Protein: 3.1g, Carbs: 47,6g, Fats: 1.6g

ADDITIONAL TITLES FROM THIS AUTHOR

70 Effective Meal Recipes to Prevent and Solve Being Overweight: Burn Fat Fast by Using Proper Dieting and Smart Nutrition

By Joe Correa CSN

48 Acne Solving Meal Recipes: The Fast and Natural Path to Fixing Your Acne Problems in Less Than 10 Days!

By Joe Correa CSN

41 Alzheimer's Preventing Meal Recipes: Reduce or Eliminate Your Alzheimer's Condition in 30 Days or Less!

By Joe Correa CSN

70 Effective Breast Cancer Meal Recipes: Prevent and Fight Breast Cancer with Smart Nutrition and Powerful Foods

By Joe Correa CSN

Printed in Great Britain
by Amazon